BUILD A BETTER YOU

A Basis for the Wise Use of Nutritional Supplementation

Dr. Richard Brouse
Chiropractic Physician

Fifth Edition
Copyright 1995

Health Education Corporation
Clackamas, Oregon

In Appreciation

The following patients and friends have been of great support to us over the years for their invitations to speak at literally hundreds of health and nutritional meetings. Their encouragement to write this booklet is greatly appreciated

Guy & Meredith Charlebois	Ottawa, Ontario
Reuben (deceased) & Rayma Cogswell	Vancouver, Washington
Floyd & Adeline Criswell	Portland, Oregon
Harvey Dennison	Clifton, New Jersey
Glenn Denune (deceased)	Olathe, Kansas
Ron & Lois Hanby	Tacoma, Washington
Gean Hemming	Ottawa, Ontario
Lee & Linda Hershberger	Enumclaw, Washington
Ed & Geri Huisman	Galt, California
Ian & Marianne Kennedy	Vancouver, British Columbia
Larry & Lois Kendel	Lloydminster, Saskatchewan
Murray & Shirley Lennox	Ottawa, Ontario
Mitch & Nancy Mitchell	Grass Valley, California
Jim & Martha Myers	Vancouver, Washington
Leon & Ellyn Naef	Lodi, California
Floyd & Dee Nelson	Salt Lake City, Utah
Herbert & Lois Pattison	Red Deer, Alberta
Marcel Poiron	Winnipeg, Manitoba
Rosie Ruther	Colorado Springs, Colorado
Jo Tonita	Vancouver, British Columbia
John Twelker	Kaneohe, Hawaii
Ivan & Martha Willmore	Fort Erie, Ontario

Without their support we would never have had the privilege to meet so many wonderful people. I am very thankful for their advice in preparing this guide.

TABLE OF CONTENTS

BASIC PRINCIPLES

One out of every three Americans will develop cancer in their lifetime. One out of every two have cardiovascular disease. One out of every nine children attend special education classes because they cannot keep up in the conventional classroom. Government studies tell us that eighty percent of all illness could be prevented or reduced by improving nutrition. Why have we become a nation of overweight and over fed observers instead of active participants in our own health? Let us look at some of the causes and what we can do to improve the situation.

Our great-great grandparents had a lifestyle that most people today do not - their daily activities included a great deal of exercise. Earning a living, caring for a home and going to and from school without the labor-saving devices we have today allowed them to earn and burn about double the calories we now require. By eating more food to do more physical activity, it was possible to get all of the needed micro nutrients and fiber from their daily diet. For most Americans, those days will never return. Because of our sedentary lifestyle, we have less demand for calories, but we still need the same 55 known essential nutrients found in food. This shift in lifestyle has opened the door for modern illness produced from suboptimal nutrition. As we enter the 21st Century, nutrition related diseases threaten the quality of life for every person. As Dr. Roger Williams stated in his book <u>Nutrition Against Disease</u>, *"It is the paradox of modern man to supplement his diet or suffer from chronic degenerative diseases."*

Reduced food quality is another factor contributing to chronic degenerative disease. Food additives, chemical fertilizers and pesticides that did not exist 100 years ago, are finding their way into our diet with accumulative detrimental affects. Literally hundreds of substances such as Red Dye #2, DDT and chloroform are removed from the food and cosmetic *safe* list each year, as adverse affects become apparent. Until these additives have stood the test of time and are known to be safe, the prudent course is to avoid them entirely.

Of all the known inhibitors of nutrition, prescription drugs are among the worst. If this statement seems controversial to you, take a quick scan of the Physicians Desk Reference describing side effects of the various drugs. In the words of one pharmacist, *"I do not know of a single drug which does not affect the absorption, utilization or loss of some nutrient."* Seldom do doctors take the time to inform their patients of the known adverse nutritional effects caused by antibiotics, anti-depressants or diuretics, to name a few. When an individual is taking several drugs, these deficiencies are compounded resulting in syndromes which defy simple diagnosis. The recent discovery that simple aspirin produces the childhood illness Reyes syndrome has made consumers more wary of drug advertising promises.

Increased nutrient requirements during times of stress are well documented in the scientific literature. In his book, The Stress of Life, Hans Selye, M.D. describes how the arousal of our body's survival instincts leads to the release of *adaptogen* hormones such as endorphins and prostaglandins. These hormones prompt sudden shifts in body chemistry, that can produce symptoms such as insomnia, localized pain, increased heart rate, labored breathing, and increased blood cholesterol. When the stress persists, chronic nutritional deficiencies will appear.

In today's high stress environment, time has become our adversary. Before the invention of electric lighting, our ancestors structured their lives in harmony with the cycle of day and night. While modern inventions offer enormous benefit, *conveniences* such as all night shopping are a barometer of just how stressful our lives have become. The future promises to be even more challenging. Change is inevitable! - Survival is essential! - Improvement is optional! This book is your resource to cope with this change and we encourage you to make the commitment to *Build a Better You*.

NOTE

Your health status today is the result of genetics, diet, accidents, stress, and pollution - but mostly, your life-style. The information contained in this booklet is not designed to treat disease or cure any illness, but rather to help you learn how disease may originate from nutritional deficiencies. As in other disciplines, prevention is wiser than treatment - and less costly in most cases. We do not guarantee any particular health benefit beyond that of better health awareness. By learning to listen to your body more precisely, you are taking responsibility for your own health.

The recommendations in this booklet are the things which a doctor expects you to be doing on your own. The information you obtain will help you - and your doctor - learn how to be more responsive to your unique biochemical needs. It is our hope that this information will start to *Build A Better You* today.

Natures Natural Medicines

The following outline briefly introduces the uses for nutritional supplementation for conditions that we have observed in our own clinic. Each statement is condensed from our clinical files and is not construed to be a treatment per se, but a preventive formula. It is also useful as a guideline for those beginning to use nutritional supplements. I have tried to write in a way that most people can understand and use this information. I have not tried to rewrite the scientific literature, but instead attempted to present the subject in a concise and convenient form. Most of this information can be confirmed by visiting a good agricultural or medical university library.

ACIDOPHILUS or BIFIDUS

Found growing in the bowel of all healthy humans, *Lactobacillus acidophilus and bifidus* cultures prevent the growth of disease-causing organisms. By producing natural antibiotics, inhibiting carcinogens and helping destroy substances that are harmful to the body, these strains of healthy microorganisms provide a necessary service to human health.

Conditions where acidophilus or bifidus may be advised in amounts beyond general recommendations (usual range - 300 to 3,600 mg per day (equivalent to 250 million to 2 billion organisms) - taken with meals):

Post antibiotic therapy - *Re-populates healthy bowel flora*
Diarrhea - *Displaces irritating foreign bacteria*
Pesticides in food - *Detoxifies many chemicals*
Eating commercial foods - *Detoxifies many additives*
Cancer of the bowel - *Detoxifies many cancer causing substances*
Toxic anxiety - *Detoxifies many neuro-toxins*
Malabsorption - *Increases availability of many trace nutrients*
Foul odor flatulence - *Displaces many fermenting bacteria*
Recurrent indigestion - *Increases digestion and absorption*
Yeast infections - *Inhibits the growth of yeast, mold and fungus in the bowel*
Colitis - *Controls secondary infection*
Hyperlipidemia - *Helps normalize blood lipids*
Taking prescription drugs - *Reduces side effects of nutrient malabsorption*

ALFALFA (Medicago sativa)

Alfalfa is one of nature's most nutritious green plants. Alfalfa leaves have a consistently high level of available minerals, protein and enzymes. It is a truly marvelous herb and food supplement. When selecting a brand, choose sources that are organically grown and harvested at peak maturity.

Conditions where alfalfa may be advised in amounts beyond general recommendations (usual range - 3 to 60 tablets per day):

Reduced kidney function - *Acts as a diuretic*
General inflammatory conditions - *Having high chlorophyll content it acts to reduce the effects of inflammatory endorphins*
Trace mineral deficiencies - *Having deep tap roots that penetrate soils often unavailable to other plants, it contains many trace minerals*
Mild digestive disorders - *Possesses three classes of enzymes for proteins, fats and carbohydrates*
Tissue water retention - *Increases kidneys filtration rate*
Elevated blood sodium levels - *Excellent source of potassium which counteracts the effects of sodium*
Slow tissue healing - *Possesses the hormone alantoin, speeds up healing*
General body odor - *Chlorophyll is natures deodorizer*
Skin blemishes and recurring rashes - *Mild antibiotic effect toward pathogenic bacteria*
High blood pressure - *Provides magnesium and potassium which relaxes arterial muscles*
Certain colon conditions - *Adds fiber, chlorophyll & vitamin K*
Ulcers - *heals damaged mucous forming cells in stomach*
Hemorrhage - *contains vitamin K which promotes normal clotting*
Diabetes - *mineral content increases insulin efficiency*
Fungal Infections - *contains anti-fungal ingredients*
Acidosis - *produces alkaline reaction in blood*
Liver Toxicity - *detoxifies liver by stimulating bile flow*
Low resistance to infections - *Enhances helper cell count in blood*
Prenatal and lactating mothers - *Good protein and calcium source*
Stiff joints - *Possesses "Anti-stiffness factor" - yet unidentified*

5

Reduce congestion the sweet way.

ANISE (Pimpinella anisum)

A sweet tasting herb used in combination with less tasteful herbs to promote detoxification.

Conditions where anise may be advised in amounts beyond general recommendations (usual range - 3 to 6 tablets per day in hot water as a tea):

Enuresis - *acts as a diuretic*
Bowel Gas - *reduces bowel flatulence*
Lung Congestion - *reduces congestion by thinning mucous*
Children's Colds - *reduces fever and congestion*

Do you have energy to soar with the eagles?

B COMPLEX FORMULA

B complex is a naturally balanced nutritional yeast formula of all 22 known (and probably some remaining unknown) B factors, whose primary function is to enhance energy production and nervous system function in cells. When selecting a brand, choose a formula with at least 100% and not more than 450% of the RDA of each B vitamin component.

Conditions where a B-complex formula may be advised in amounts beyond general recommendations (usual range - 3 to 20 tablets or capsules per day - enough to keep your urine an orange-yellow color):

General fatigue - *Essential for cellular energy production*
Loss of appetite - *Stimulates hypothalamus for hunger and satiety*
Sleep disorders - *Necessary for production of sleep inducing hormones*
Nervousness - *Raises activation threshold of nerves*
Anxiety - *Reduces adrenaline release*
Depression - *Regulates normal anti-depressant hormone production*
Digestive disorders - *Regulates digestive hormone release*
Weight gain or loss - *Stabilizes fat metabolism*

Grossly imbalanced diet - *Provides most often missed dietary nutrients*
Taking prescription drugs - *Replaces nutrients lost from side effects*
Hypoglycemia - *Allows adrenal-pancreas-liver balance of blood sugar*
Alcoholism - *Reduces desire for refined sugars*
High Stress - *Replaces nutrients lost from excessive loss through kidneys*

Do the bright lights of driving bother your eyes?

BETA-CAROTENE

Now known to be necessary for prevention of many illnesses, this vegetable form of pro-vitamin A is essential for optimum health.

Conditions where Beta-carotene may be advised in amounts beyond general recommendations (usual range - 10,000 to 80,000 IU's per day - enough to produce carrot color in palms of hands and soles of feet):

Difficulty with night vision - *Source of vitamin A for vision at night*
General inflammatory conditions - *Anti-oxidant effect on free radicals*
Recurrent viral infections - *anti-viral*
Slow wound healing - *Promotes epithelial tissue growth*
Dry and rough skin - *Reduces effects of UV light from the sun*
Frequent urinary infections - *Promotes healthy mucous membranes in bladder and urethra*
Sinusitis - *Promotes healing of mucous membranes after infection*
Allergies and asthma - *Reduces damage to mucous membranes caused by histamine release*
Skin blemishes - *Nourishes epithelium to resist infection*
Low blood pressure - *Strengthens contractibility of heart muscle*
Colitis - *Promotes healing and reduces scarring*
Low resistance to infections - *Raises killer cell activity*
Diverticulitis - *Strengthens bowel muscles and mucous membranes*
Repeated middle ear infections - *Prevents inflammation of the eustachian tubes due to allergies or sensitivities*

Eye health at its best.

BILBERRY (Vaccinum myrtillus)

This shrubby plant produces succulent fruit closely related to blueberry and cranberry. Recent research shows remarkable healing benefits for certain eye conditions as well as other general qualities.

Conditions where bilberry may be advised in amounts beyond general recommendations (usual range - 3 to 12 tablets per day or in hot water as a tea):

Glaucoma - *reduces pressure in the eye*
Cataracts - *improves circulation and reduces lens opacity*
Infections - *has antibiotic properties*
Diarrhea - *reduces irritation from virus and bacterial exotoxins*
Bad Breath - *chewing the dried berries reduces bacterial
    mouth odors*
Stress Anorexia - *helps restore appetite*
Bowel Gas - *controls gas causing bacteria in the lower bowel*

A healer and tissue conditioner.

BLUE MELVA FLOWER (Malva sylvestris)

A lowly scrubby plant which often grows in waste ground, rubbish dumps and along fence rows, it has remarkable healing properties.

Conditions where blue melva flower may be advised in amounts beyond general recommendations (usual range - 3 to 12 tablets per day or in hot water as a tea):

Muscle fatigue - *acts as an astringent to tighten tissue*
Cough - *reduces irritation to throat*
Hoarseness - *relieves vocal chord inflammation*
Laryngitis - *reduces inflammation of throat*
Open Wounds - *reduces swelling, promotes healing when
    used as a wash*
Irritable Bowel - *reduces bowel inflammation*
Bronchitis - *soothes irritated bronchial tubes*
Emphysema - *reduces congestion and thick mucous*

Clean from the inside out.

BUCKTHORN BARK (Rhamnus frangula)

A relative of Cascara sagrada, Buckthorn has been used for centuries for detoxification and as a colon tonic.

Conditions where buckthorn may be advised in amounts beyond general recommendations (usual range - 3 to 12 tablets per day or in hot water as a tea):

Constipation - *gently stimulates normal bowel motility*
Cancer - *contains tumor preventive glycosides*
Water Retention - *acts as a safe diuretic*
Gall Bladder Disease - *reduces irritation caused by inflamed gall bladder*
Lead Toxicity - *detoxifies liver*
Hemorrhoids - *reduces swelling and itching*

Are you having muscle cramps?

CALCIUM

Calcium is a natural mineral the body needs for bones and many other body functions. It requires a minimal amount of stomach acid for ionization and absorption.

Conditions where calcium may be advised in amounts beyond general recommendations (usual range - 150 to 1,500 mg per day):

Dairy product avoidance - *offsets calcium deficiency*
Post exercise muscle cramps or spasms - *relaxes over-stressed muscles*
Allergic rhinitis (hay fever) - *reduces hyperimmune response*
Taking prescription drugs - *offsets drug induced deficiencies*
Menstrual cramping - *relaxes smooth muscles*
Prenatal muscle cramps - *needed for proper muscle relaxation*

CALCIUM MAGNESIUM

A formula of calcium blended with magnesium, phosphorus, vitamin D and trace nutrients is essential for the maintenance of healthy bones and teeth. When selecting a brand, the calcium:magnesium ratio should be between 2:1 to 1:1.

Conditions where calcium magnesium may be advised in amounts beyond general recommendations (usual range - 150 to 1500 mg of the calcium component per day):

Dental bone loss - *prevents resorption of bone*
Rapid bone growth and healing - *provides proper building blocks*
Repetitive motion arthritic pain - *decreases stress on bone and connective tissue*
Osteoporosis - *necessary for bone integrity*
Menstrual cramps - *needed for proper muscle relaxation*
Headaches - *reduces vascular tension*
Taking prescription drugs - *offsets drug induced deficiencies*
Prenatal calcium deficiency - *provides for added need during pregnancy*

Calm those nerves.

CHAMOMILE (Maticaria chamomilla)

Known for centuries to be a good nerve tonic, this flowered herb is used widely through out the world.

Conditions where chamomile may be advised in amounts beyond general recommendations (usual range - 3 to 9 tablets per day in hot water as a tea):

Nervousness - *relaxes nervous system*
Insomnia - *releases serotonin from brain*
Poor Appetite - *stimulates hypothalamus to taste*
Indigestion - *relieves gastric upset*
Cystitis - *relieves bladder muscles preventing infections*
Colds - *reduces muscle aches from virus*
Asthma - *relieves bronchial spasm*
Colitis - *reduces inflammation and irritation to bowel mucosa*

10

Diverticulosis - *mild laxative effect reduces bowel pressures*
Fever - *reduces pyrogenic effect to nervous system*
Headaches - *calms neck muscles reducing vascular back-pressure*
Hemorrhoids - *increases bowel circulation*
Muscle cramps - *calms irritated muscles*
Rheumatism - *reduces inflammatory hormones in muscles*
Arthritis - *reduces inflammatory hormones in joints*
Worm Parasites - *sedates round worms in bowel causing expulsion*
Jaundice - *reduces blood circulating bilirubin*

Reduce your pain.

CULVER'S ROOT (Leptandra virginica)

Used as a general pain reliever and digestive aid without side effects, this herb has a history dating back to the Roman legionnaires.

Conditions where culver's root may be advised in amounts beyond general recommendations (usual range - 3 to 12 tablets per day or in hot water as a tea):

Indigestion - *reduces stomach distress*
Hepatitis - *detoxifies liver from virus infection and food poisoning*
Jaundice - *increases bile flow from gall bladder*
Headaches - *decreases neck muscle tension*
Bursitis - *relieves shoulder pain*

EPA

Deep ocean fish have a unique oil which is amazing in its ability to help reduce the effects of stress. EPA is important in keeping serum lipids at a healthy level. EPA is usually paired with DHA, a related fish oil, in an EPA:DHA ratio of 3:1

Conditions where EPA may be advised in amounts beyond general recommendations (usual range - 180 to 1800 mg of the EPA component per day):

Heart disorders - *reduces work demand on heart*
Circulation problems - *increases flow rate in small blood vessels*
Elevated cholesterol - *increases HDL, decreases LDL fractions*
Elevated triglycerides - *improves liver metabolism of fats*
Heavy stress - *produces anti-stress hormones*

Do you protect your immune system?

ECHINACEA (Echinacea angustfolia & purpurea)

Indigenous to North America, early settlers were taught by friendly Indians to use Echinacea for many conditions. As a blood and lymphatic detoxifier, antiseptic, anti-viral and analgesic, the root of the Purple Coneflower was used more broadly by the plains Indians than any other herb. Prolonged use of more than several months reduces its effectiveness.

Conditions where echinacea may be advised in amounts beyond general recommendations (usual range - 3 to 12 tablets per day as a poultice or in hot water as a tea):

Tonsillitis - *reduces swelling of lymphatic tissue in tonsils*
Tooth Aches - *when taken as a tea or applied as a poultice reduces pain, inflammation and infection*
Sore Throat - *soothes irritated mucous membranes of throat*
Insect Bites - *prevents itching, swelling and infection*
Insect Repellent - *secreted through pores and discourages insects*
Animal Bites - *prevents infection from pathogenic bacteria found on pets claws and teeth*

Snake Bites - *as a poultice, resists hemolytic and neurological poison reactions*

Fevers - *neutralizes pyrogenic effect in the body to reduce high temperature*

Chronic Infections - *mobilizes immune system to overcome infections*

Chest Congestion - *reduces and thins mucous*

Eczema - *reduces skin sensitivity caused from allergies and sensitivities*

Poisonous Plants - *reduces immune response to poison ivy, oak & sumac*

Low Blood Pressure - *one of the few substances known to normalize blood pressure when low*

Cancer - *mobilizes immune factors to fight and prevent cancer*

Virus Infections - *prevents and speeds healing of flu and colds*

Childhood Immunizations - *prevents serum reaction and complications to the immune system*

Toxicity - *enhanced recovery from food & chemical poisoning*

Burns - *reduces pain, inflammation and secondary infections*

Heat Sensitivity - *conditions against hot or cold injuries*

Decongest and breath freely again.

EUCALYPTUS (Eucalyptus globulus)

This pleasant aromatic leaf is used to promote healing and enhance the beneficial effects of other herbs.

Conditions where eucalyptus may be advised in amounts beyond general recommendations (usual range - 3 to 12 tablets per day or in hot water as a tea or in steam):

Sinus Congestion - *thins sinus mucous and promotes drainage*

Sore Throat - *soothes irritated mucous membranes*

Cough - *suppresses cough reflex*

Colds - *mild anti-viral effect*

Joint Aches - *relieves pain from mild arthritis*

Muscle Pains - *soothes overworked or injured muscles*

Get the system going.

FENNEL (Foeniculum vulgare)

A sweet herb used to add a pleasant taste to other herbal preparations while increasing energy and improving digestion.

Conditions where fennel may be advised in amounts beyond general recommendations (usual range - 3 to 12 tablets per day in hot water as a tea):

Appetite - *suppresses appetite*
Eye Irritations - *soothes irritated eye membranes*
Liver congestion - *Increases bile production*
Decreased kidney function - *increases filtration rate*
Intestinal gas - reduces *flatulence*
GI distress - *reduces irritation to mucous membranes*
Gout - *reduces uric acid*
Cancer chemotherapy & radiation - *promotes detoxification*

Are you using nature's antibiotic?

GARLIC (Allium sativa)

Garlic is a supplement which thins the blood, increases nutrient absorption, kills viruses and prevents bacteria from growing. When garlic is blended with vitamin E and vitamin A and the herb rosemary, the usual strong taste and after effects are lessened.

Conditions where garlic may be advised in amounts beyond general recommendations (usual range - 3 to 12 tablets per day or in hot water as a tea):

Recurrent viral infections - *anti-viral*
Colitis - *anti-inflammatory*
Malabsorption - *increases digestive juice release*
Upper respiratory infections - *anti-bacterial*
High blood pressure - *anti-hypertensive*
Smoking - *detoxification*
Intermittent claudication - *increases capillary circulation*
Sinus and nasal congestion -*decongestant*
Hyperglycemia - *lowers elevated blood sugar*
Chronic bronchitis - *anti-inflammatory*
Post surgical recovery - *speeds tissue healing*

Atherosclerosis - *dilates small blood vessels*
Blood clots - *prevents clotting*
Hyperlipidemia - *dissolves fatty deposits and thins blood*
Fatty degenerative liver - *speeds liver healing*

Do you have a sensitive or queasy stomach?

GINGER (Zingiber officinale)

Oriental history depicts ginger as the most widely used herb offering relief from many conditions because of its ability to increase the body's basal metabolism. Used raw from fresh cut ginger root or the dried concentrate, ginger offers safe relief from many conditions treatable only by dangerous drugs.

Conditions where ginger may be advised in amounts beyond general recommendations (usual range - 1 to 9 tablets per day as a hot tea):

Menstrual Cramps - *reduces uterine congestion and stimulates calcium absorption*
Nausea - *reduces effects of rich food or chemical irritation in the stomach*
Morning Sickness - *as a first beverage in the morning, reduces nausea before meals*
Digestive Aid - *reduces excess stomach acid which causes gastritis*
Dysentery - *reduces effects of bacterial exotoxins in the bowel*
Food Poisoning - *effectively used to treat mushroom or ergot toxins*
Motion Sickness - *relieves nervous reflex between stomach and brain to calm sea or car sickness*
Common Cold - *sipped every hour, greatly speeds recovery*
Circulation - *taken orally or ground and put in a bath, the lasting effects on capillaries reduces pain and stiffness of muscles*

Most prized of all herbs.

GINSENG (Panax Ginseng)

Ancient Chinese legends say that ginseng was made specifically to help mankind with a whole host of health problems. With roots growing two feet in length and divided at the end to resemble the lower torso, the plant takes on the shape of a human. The word *"panacea"* is the Latin enhancement of Panax - *"used to treat everything."* The active components are a family of phytochemicals called *"ginsenosides"* which have not been able to be synthetically duplicated. Wealthy Orientals still prize ginseng as a daily tonic to promote vigor and vitality, as well as extend life. Fresh or dried, then later made into a tea, ginseng is cultivated for its revitalizing properties.

Conditions where ginseng may be advised in amounts beyond general recommendations (usual range 3 tablets dissolved in hot water after each meal):

Fatigue - *revives energy after strenuous exercise*
Nervousness - *calms nerves*
Lack of Libido - *revives sex drive in men and women*
Infections - *builds immune factors including interferon*
Memory - *increases recall of details*
Concentration - *maintains ability to focus attention*
Pain - *reduces musculo-skeletal pain*
Toxicity - *helps secretory function of kidneys and gall bladder*
Chemical Dependence - *reduces addiction craving*
Circulation - *improves capillary permeability*
PMS - *helps reduce tension, anxiety, depression and muscle pain*
Low Body Temperature - *promotes higher basal metabolic rate*

Are the stresses of life causing hormone
imbalance and elevated blood fats?

GLA

Gamma Linoleic Acid or GLA is an oil from plants such as Evening Primrose or Borage seed which provides a boost to the hormone producing organs of the body. GLA provides a support during stressful times to prevent distress.

Conditions where GLA may be advised in amounts beyond general recommendations (usual range - 200 to 2000 mg per day):

Hormone imbalances - *minimizes fluctuations due to nutrient deficiency*
Circulation problems - *helps prostaglandin regulation of circulation*
Adaptation to stress - *calms nervous release of adrenaline*
Elevated blood fats - *overcomes fat reduction of GLA synthesis*
Premenstrual syndrome (PMS) - *reduces headaches*
Skin eruptions and dryness - *helps synthesis of natural skin oils for healing*
Menopause - *helps spare body estrogen stores*

Are you carrying toxins in your body?

HERBAL LAXATIVE FORMULA

Many people find a natural gastro-intestinal purgative, containing soluble fiber and herbs (such as senna leaf, licorice root, alfalfa, fennel seed, anise root and rhubarb root) helps them with bowel cleansing and regularity. An herbal laxative formula functions to prevent the accumulation of metabolic wastes, which in turn limits cellular damage and promotes blood and cellular cleansing.

Conditions where an herbal laxative formula may be advised in amounts beyond general recommendations (usual range - 1 to 4 tablets or capsules with meals, before bed or as a tea):

Infections & simple acne - *reduces body bacterial count*
Unpleasant body odor - *detoxifies body waste*
Agricultural chemical exposure - *removes toxic substances from bowel before absorption*

17

Surgically induced lazy bowel - *stimulates exercising of bowel muscles*
Bowel transit times beyond 12 hours - *speeds transit time and reduces bowel pressure*
Influenza - *helps the body remove toxins*
Taking prescription drugs - *removes toxic drug byproducts*
Blood cleanser - *prevents accumulation of metabolic waste products*

Soothe irritated membranes.

HOREHOUND (Marrubium vulgare)

This European herb has been used for centuries to treated chest and throat related illnesses.

Conditions where Horehound may be advised in amounts beyond general recommendations (usual range - 3 to 6 tablets per day or in hot water as a tea or as a syrup or candy):

Cough - *reduces cough reflex*
Colds - *reduces sneezing reflex*
Asthma - *relieves bronchial irritation from air born allergens*
Jaundice - *promotes normal liver function*
Sore Throat - *soothes irritated mucous membranes*
Intestinal Gas - *reduces flatulence*
Bowel Parasites - *discourages round worms in the bowel*

A folk remedy that works!

HYSSOP (Hyssopus officinale)

This Biblical herb has had an almost superstitious application for wound healing, infection prevention and cleansing. Science has shown that it harbors natural penicillin growing on its leaves. Hyssop is often used with other herbs and teas to enhance their properties.

Conditions where Hyssop may be advised in amounts beyond general recommendations (usual range - 1 to 6 tablets per day):

Constipation - *promotes bowel regularity*
Dysentery - *controls the growth of pathogenic bacteria*

Slow Wound Healing - *promotes healing by inhibiting harmful bacteria*
Bowel Infections - *helps to restore friendly bacteria*
Detoxification - *inhibits putrefactive bacteria and enhances bowel cleansing*

Are you providing proper care and feeding to your immune system?

IMMUNE FORMULA

Proper function of our immune system is essential if we want to stay healthy. Factors known to enhance immune function include: beta-carotene, vitamins C, E, B_6, B_{12}, folic acid, iron, copper, selenium, zinc, echinacea, and thymus.

Conditions where an immune formula may be advised in amounts beyond general recommendations (usual range - 1 to 6 tablets or capsules per day):

Repeated viral infections - *promotes interferon production*
Cancer prevention - *detoxifies carcinogens*
Skin and cuticle infections - *boosts lymphocyte aggressiveness*
Boils - *promotes infection resistant skin*
Pre-immunization - *reduces risk of hyper-immune response*
Recurring respiratory infections - *improves lymphatic flow to lungs and bronchi*
Sore throat - *improves resistance to pharyngeal infections*
Animal handling - *prevents secondary infections from small scratches*
Allergies - *promotes normal immune response*
Auto-immune illnesses - *reduces over-active immune response*
Following blood transfusions - *prevents minor incompatibility reactions*

Are you feeling tired or cold and looking pale?

IRON

Iron is an essential component of red blood cells and is needed for cellular respiration. Some forms of iron can cause constipation. Vegetable based iron supplements are usually less constipating and iron should be paired with vitamin C to enhance absorption.

New research points to a possible link between too much iron and increased risk of heart disease, so high doses of iron should only be taken under a doctor's supervision.

Conditions where iron may be advised in amounts beyond general recommendations (usual range - 18 to 30 mg per day):

Iron deficiency anemia - *taken with vitamin C, is most easily absorbed*
Previous stomach surgery - *offsets poor iron absorption due to lack of binding factors*
Malabsorption syndrome - *easily absorbed when taken with food*
Teenage girls - *offsets usual avoidance of iron rich foods*
Aspirin toxicity - *replaces iron lost from bowel irritation*
Prescription drugs - *offsets loss from drug side effects*
Prenatal anemia - *fetal growth may be reducing the mother's iron supply*

How do we prevent thick blood?

LECITHIN

Lecithin is a natural emulsifier and absorptive aid for fat soluble nutrients such as vitamins A, D, E, K and the essential fatty acids. It is also an excellent source of choline, inositol and other neuro-transmitter (sleep inducing) hormones. Look for a product with a choline:inositol ratio of approximately 3:2.

Conditions where lecithin may be advised in amounts beyond general recommendations (usual range - 500 to 5000 mg per day):

Post gall bladder surgery - *assists emulsification of essential fat soluble nutrients*

Elevated serum cholesterol - *converts to good (HDL) cholesterol*
Gallstone tendencies - *dissolves cholesterol containing stones*
Insomnia - *assists neuro-transmitter production in brain*
Viral infections - *aids in immune function*
Nervousness - *relaxes nervous system*
Learning disabilities - *enhances attention span*
Early senility - *improves brain circulation*
Liver cirrhosis - *protects against further liver damage*
Chemical sensitivities - *detoxifies through liver*

More than just a taste treat!

LICORICE (Glycyrrhiza glabra)

The sweet taste of this herb has made it ideal for flavoring soft drinks, candy and tea. Containing a compound called glycyrrhizin, licorice has many beneficial affects to the body.

Conditions where Licorice may be advised in amounts beyond general recommendations (usual range - 3 to 12 tablets per day as a poultice, syrup or in hot water as a tea):

Hypoglycemia - *helps regulate blood sugar through adrenal relaxation*
Bronchitis - *reduces bronchiospasm by restoring tissue catecholamines*
Colitis - *lengthens life of intestinal cells and improves micro-circulation*
Diverticulosis - *improves quality of bowel mucous thus reduces bowel pressure*
Gastritis - *increases amount of mucous secreting cells in the stomach which protects against hydrochloric acid*
Stress - *promotes adrenal gland function*
Colds - *stimulates production of interferon*
Nausea - *desensitizes stomach nausea receptors*
Inflammation - *neutralizes endorphins which cause tissue swelling*

Do you have trouble swallowing tablets?

LIQUID VITAMIN/MINERAL SUPPLEMENT

Liquid multiple vitamin/mineral products are helpful for individuals such as infants or the elderly who have difficulty swallowing tablets or capsules. When selecting a brand, choose a product with approximately 50-100% of the RDA of each of the nutrient components in one teaspoonful. (Note: Liquid vitamin/mineral supplements will be lacking in vitamin C, calcium and other nutrients.)

Conditions where a liquid vitamin/mineral supplement may be advised in amounts beyond general recommendations (usual range - 1 to 2 teaspoons with meals:

Iron or folic acid deficiency - *provides most common deficient nutrient devoid in foods*
Malabsorption - *bypasses need for solid form disintegration*
General fatigue - *rapid absorption produces rapid energy return*
Difficulty in swallowing pills - *provides nutrition in liquid form*
Gastric Surgery - *minimizes stress to stomach and bowel recovery*
Prenatal and nursing mothers - *rapidly rebuilds nutrient pool and maintains optimum blood levels*

Soothes mucous membranes.

MARSHMALLOW ROOT (Althaea officinalis)

The mucilaginous gel from this plant has been used internally and externally for a broad assortment of illnesses.

Conditions where Marshmallow may be advised in amounts beyond general recommendations (usual range - 3 to 9 tablets per day or in hot water as a tea or poultice):

Pain - *general pain reduction*
Coughs - *suppresses reflex*
Hoarseness - *reduces inflamed vocal cords*
Tonsillitis - *clears tonsil inflammation*
Stings - *pain from wasp and bee stings are quickly relieved*

Inflammation - *reduces swelling in irritated eyes and skin*
Mouth - *reduces swollen Abscesses*

Are you balancing your minerals?

MULTIPLE MINERAL COMPLEX

A multiple mineral complex containing naturally occurring calcium, magnesium, zinc, manganese and chromium is essential for enzyme and hormone activation.

Conditions where a multiple mineral complex may be advised in amounts beyond general recommendations (usual range - 1 to 6 tablets or capsules per day):

Familial osteoporosis tendencies - *Effectively retards bone loss in small framed people*
Post menopausal bone loss - *Prevents decalcification of bone*
Premenstrual syndrome *(PMS)* - *Combines effective calcium and magnesium with essential trace minerals for hormone synthesis*
Menstrual cramps - *needed for proper muscle tonicity*

Do you have energy highs or lows?

MULTIPLE VITAMIN/MINERAL SUPPLEMENT

A multiple vitamin/mineral supplement contains cofactors and coenzymes which enhance protein utilization. Science has discovered many known nutrients and undoubtedly this process will continue as nutritional research progresses. Multiple vitamin/mineral supplements that contain whole food sources of nutrients may contain vitamins which science has not yet discovered. A multiple vitamin/mineral supplement works best when used in conjunction with a high quality protein powder. When selecting a brand, choose a product with at least 50% of the RDA of all essential vitamins and minerals in one tablet or capsule.

To test the quality of the product you are considering, see how long it takes for the supplement to break down in a glass of water. If it does not break down within 20 to 40 minutes, you may have difficulty digesting and absorbing the nutrients.

Conditions where a multiple vitamin/mineral supplement may be advised in amounts beyond general recommendations (usual range - 1 to 3 tablets or capsules with each meal per day):

Failure to thrive - *promotes anabolism (healthy growth)*
Prenatal vitamin - *provides for the added needs during pregnancy*
Nursing mothers - *provides for added needs during breast feeding*
Bone wasting - *Stabilizes bone metabolism*
Poor hair & nail growth - *activates protein synthesis*
Weight loss or weight gain - *normalizes body size*
Prescription drug induced nutrient deficiencies - *replaces lost nutrients due to interactions*
Chemical dependency withdrawal - *replaces neglected nutrients*

Having digestive problems?

PEPPERMINT (Mentha Piperita)

Known for its odiferous oil, peppermint has medicinal properties which have been recognized since the time of ancient Egypt. Acting to release parasympathetic nerve hormones in the body, peppermint has a soothing and healing effect on many systems. When mixed with other herbal teas, peppermint assists their absorption and enhances their effectiveness.

Conditions where peppermint tea may be advised in amounts beyond general recommendations (usual range - 3 tablets dissolved in hot water with meals):

Indigestion - *releases stomach gastrin to normalize digestion*
Food Allergies - *reduces bowel inflammation and irritability*
Irritable Bowel - *restores normal permeability to bowel mucosa*
Diarrhea - *improves bowel absorption slowing transit time*
Gastric Ulcers - *reduces hydrochloric acid production between meals*
Sore Throat - *soothes irritated mucosa tissue of throat*
Stress Reaction - *calms sympathetic nerves associated with stress*
Abdominal Cramping - *relaxes smooth muscle contractions*
Bowel Gas - *promotes digestion thus reducing gas formation*
Constipation - *relaxes tense or spastic bowel muscles*

Headaches - *relieves cerebral vascular and muscular tension*
Bad Breath - *neutralizes mouth odors*

Are you meeting your daily protein needs?

PROTEIN POWDER

Proper burning of dietary calories in an efficient manner is essential for achieving peak conditioning. Protein powder provides fiber, protein, vitamins and minerals to achieve this process. It is low in fat, and helps active individuals keep their energy level up. When selecting a brand, choose a protein powder with a PER (Protein Efficiency Ratio) of at least 2.5.

Conditions where protein powder may be advised in amounts beyond general recommendations (usual range - 1 to 3 tablespoons with water, juice, on cereal or combined with recipes):

Calorie limiting diets - *high nutrient density*
Certain forms of colitis - *prevents irritation from allergens*
Diabetes - *helps to stabilize blood sugar*
Habitual eating disorders - *satisfies basic nutrient needs*
Hypoglycemia - *helps to stabilize blood sugar*
Light meal replacement - *less calories per total nutrient dense serving*
Post-natal and nursing mothers - *optimum protein to calorie ratio*
Protein sparing weight control programs - *prevents muscle wasting while burning fat*
Rapid growth spurts - *satisfies needs of rapid growing youthful bodies*
Recovery from surgery - *provides building blocks for rapid recovery*
Therapeutic weight reduction - *prevents muscle wasting while speeding weight loss*
Vegetarianism - *provides most often neglected trace nutrients in vegetarian diet*
Weight training or weight reduction - *combined with exercise, maximizes reduction of fat while maintaining muscle mass*

Do you get all of the roughage you need from your diet?

PSYLLIUM FIBER

Soluble and insoluble fiber is needed to remove accumulating toxins from the body. Psyllium fiber helps rehabilitate and condition the heart and associated blood vessels and is a convenient way to get the bulk back into our diet.

Conditions where psyllium fiber may be advised in amounts beyond general recommendations (usual range - 1 to 3 tablespoons per day):

Angina - *removes pain causing auto-toxins*
Chronic constipation - *increases peristaltic action*
Elevated cholesterol - *prevents fat absorption*
Hemorrhoids - *reduces bowel pressure*
Hypertension - *reduces hypertensive bacterial wastes*
Irregular heart rhythms - *reduces heart irritants*
Ischemic heart disease - *reduces demand on oxygen depleting detoxification process*
Liver Disorders - *helps remove the toxic load on the liver*
Post heart attack - *reduces stress on heart by minimizing fat accumulation*
Stroke - *reduces insoluble waste in blood*

Good for more than pie!

RHUBARB ROOT (Rheum palmatum)

This abundant herb hosts a number of medicinal properties differing from its toxic leaf.

Conditions where Rhubarb Root may be advised in amounts beyond general recommendations (usual range - 3 to 12 tablets per day or in hot water as a tea):

Colitis - *reduces irritation to mucous membranes of lower bowel*
Liver Congestion - *promotes liver cleansing*
Headaches - *blocks endorphin effect on the brain similar to aspirin*
Diarrhea - *inhibits growth of dysentery causing bacteria*
Constipation - *increases lower bowel motility*

Hemorrhoids - *reduces circulatory pressure on lower bowel*
Worm Parasites - *irritates the digestive tract of round worms*
Duodenal Ulcers - *promotes healing of upper GI mucous membranes*
Gallbladder Distress - *thins bile*
Bacterial Infections - *mild antibiotic effect*

The sweetest smelling herb of all.

ROSEMARY (Rosemarinus officinalis)

Called "dew of the sea" by ancient physicians, including Hippocrates, this culinary herb was once thought to be the greatest aromatic herb in the Mediterranean area. Used effectively in repelling fleas during the Black Plague, it was also used throughout Europe to prevent other infectious disease. Many European households still grow and place rosemary twigs around the home and especially in the room of the ill.

Conditions where Rosemary may be advised in amounts beyond general recommendations (usual range - 3 to 9 tablets per day or in hot water as a tea):

Fleas - *repels biting insects*
Bad Breath - *freshens breath*
Memory - *increases brain circulation*
Cold - *promotes quick recovery from virus infections*
Headache - *reduces circulatory congestion to the brain*
Convalescence - *stimulates recuperative powers of the ill*

Keep things going.

SENNA (Cassia angustifolia)

Senna is an effective laxative for adults which stimulates upper and lower bowel motility. Total body cleansing should include this herb.

Conditions where Senna may be advised in amounts beyond general recommendations (usual range - 1 to 6 tablets per day or in hot water as a tea):

Constipation - *increases moisture content of stool and increases motility of bowel*
Intestinal Parasites - *acts as a vermifuge*
Halitosis - *reduces bad odors from bacterial and toxic substances*

"Let your food be your medicine."

SOY BEAN (Glycine max)

Used in Asia as a primary dietary protein source, the soy bean has been made into a number of useful products to aid the health of man.

Conditions where Soy may be advised as a food supplement in amounts beyond general recommendations (usual range - 3 to 12 tablespoons per day on cereal, in juice or in a fruit shake):

Morning Sickness - *reduces sensitivity to food smells and tastes during pregnancy*
Menopause - *enhances estrogen effects in receptor cells*
Hot Flashes - *helps prevent adrenal and thyroid "storms"*
PMS - *reduces aches and pains associated with menstruation*

Sweet and spicy.

SPEARMINT (Mentha spicata)

Milder than peppermint, this herb sweetens many other herbal formulas.

Conditions where Spearmint may be advised in amounts beyond general recommendations (usual range - 3 to 12 tablets per day or in hot water as a tea):

Bladder Infections - *relieves irritation from bacterial cystitis*
Bad Breath - *sweetens breath*
Colds - *reduces congestion*
Pneumonia - *used to reduce infusion of fluid in lung*
Fever - *has a cooling effect on body*
Bowel Gas - *reduces flatulence*
Nausea - *reduces gag reflex*

Mother Thyme and Father Time work together.

THYME (Thymus vulgaris)

This commonly occurring highly aromatic window box plant has an excellent reputation for flavoring stew, soups and stuffing. It also is used extensively for women's problems, lung problems, children's infections and fevers. Thyme works best when combined with other herbs.

Conditions where an immune formula may be advised in amounts beyond general recommendations (usual range - 1 to 6 tablets or capsules per day):

Vaginitis - *soothes and cools inflamed tissue*
Parasites - *kills and repels skin and bowel microbes*
Insect Repellent - *repels biting insects*
Abscesses - *reduces swelling and infection*
Indigestion - *calms nervous or sour stomach in children*
Bad Breath - *natural deodorizer*
Sore Throat - *soothes irritated throat*
Whooping cough - *reduces coughing reflex*
Wounds - *mild antiseptic*

For rest and relaxation.

VALERIAN (Valeriana officinalis)

People who have occasional difficulty relaxing or falling to sleep will appreciate the gentle non-addictive effect valerian can provide. Used for centuries for treating traumatic pain, nervousness and general irritability, valerian has a broad reputation for helping normalize body functions.

Conditions where Valerian may be advised in amounts beyond general recommendations (usual range - 3 to 12 tablets per day in hot water or at night as a tea):

Nervousness - *restores relaxed state to central nervous system*
Ulcers - *relaxes vagus nerve stimuli*
Headaches - *relieves tension in neck and brain stem allowing normal circulation*
Colic - *reduces pain from gastric irritation*
Gas - *acts as an anti-flatulent*

Pain - *raises pain threshold from smooth and striated muscles*
Stress - *reduces nervous system tension*
Anxiety - *reduces sympathetic nerve reflex similar to anti-anxiety drugs*
Insomnia - *allows relaxation to bring on restful sleep*
Convulsions - *calms brain wave patterns*
Muscle cramps - *relaxes sympathetic nervous stimuli*
Colds - *reduces mucous*

Are you giving your white blood cells the weapons they need to fight?

VITAMIN C

Vitamin C aids in a multitude of body functions. It is a powerful immune stimulant as well as an anti-oxidant. Virtually every body function benefits from an adequate level of vitamin C. The best vitamin C supplements are made from natural sources and complexed with bioflavonoids in a 4:1 ratio.

Conditions where vitamin C may be advised in amounts beyond general recommendations (usual range - 500 to 10,000 mg per day):

Cancer prevention - *detoxifies carcinogens and extends life expectancy*
Viral infections - *increases blood interferon*
Iron deficiency anemia - *assists iron absorption*
Stress response - *calms nerves*
Mineral absorption - *assists mineral absorption*
Chronic constipation - *mild laxative*
Respiratory distress - *thins mucous*
Immunizations - *prevents hyper-immune response*
Fevers - *reduces length of fever*
Congestion - *decongestant*
Taking prescription drugs - *detoxifies many drugs*
Wound healing - *speeds tissue healing*
Muscle strains and sprains - *speeds healing of connective tissue*
Chemical sensitivity - *detoxifies sensitizing substances and boosts immune system*
Allergies - *reduces histamine release*
Headaches - *reduces vascular tension*
Insomnia - *helps release*
Body aches and pains - *anti-inflammatory*
Smoking - *detoxifies toxic gases including carbon monoxide*

Prenatal and lactating mothers - *prevents infections and enhances the babies immune system*
Preparing for and recovering from surgery - *rapid healing*
Fatigue- *boosts body energy*
Bruising easily- *maintains connective tissue integrity*
Collagen formation - *prevents tearing of capillaries*

You are breathing, but are you using your oxygen?

VITAMIN E WITH SELENIUM

Vitamin E and selenium are two powerful anti-oxidants. Together they help prevent cellular damage from harmful free radicals. When selecting a brand, choose a product with 100 to 400 IU vitamin E and 10 mcg Selenium per capsule. Vitamin E is available in water soluble and oil soluble forms. Oil soluble vitamin E can be taken internally or applied topically to the skin. When applied to injuries, such as a burn, vitamin E helps prevent scar formation. The water soluble form of vitamin E is for those who want to minimize dietary oils or have a sensitive gall bladder.

Conditions where vitamin E and selenium may be advised in amounts beyond general recommendations (usual range - 1 to 5 capsules per day):

Cancer prevention - *reduces accumulation of peroxides*
Slow wound healing - *promotes healing of skin, bowel and soft tissue*
Poor limb circulation - *increases capillary blood flow*
Low blood pressure - *improves efficiency of heart muscle*
Anemia - *protects red blood cell membranes*
Aging - *prevents oxidized fat accumulation and free radical damage*
Hormonal stabilization - *prevents hormonal storms caused by oxygen fluctuations*

ZINC

Lost in our soil due to unnatural farming methods, adequate amounts of zinc are lacking in the diets of four out of five people. Products with zinc gluconate complexed with alfalfa are a very bio-available form of zinc.

Conditions where zinc may be advised in amounts beyond general recommendations (usual range - 15 to 60 mg per day):

Skin blemishes - *promotes infection prevention and decreases acne scars*
Liver disorders - *actives over 80 known liver enzymes*
Mineral imbalances - *one of the most depleted minerals in the average diet*
Wound healing - *needed for connective tissue repair in scar tissue*
Sore throat - *inhibits viral and bacterial infections of pharynx*
Low energy - *activates ergogenic process*
Arthritis - *depleted in many types of arthritis*
Prostatitis - *promotes healthy prostate*
Cataracts - *needed for dissolving clouded lens*
White spots on nails - *common finding in zinc deficient persons*

HEALTH CARE vs. DISEASE CARE

From clinical experience, we have found that nutrients tend to work better when used together - this is called synergism. Except in a few cases, attempts to treat illness using individual nutrients usually fail. True lasting healing comes from the body's innate (natural) power to recognize, organize and fabricate a higher level of health from the molecular building blocks in food.

Prescription or over the counter drugs can never take the place of optimum nutrition. We are the largest drug consuming nation in the world, and yet we rank as one having the poorest health of all developed nations.

Drugs act by either inhibiting or stimulating the enzyme processes inside a cell. Many symptoms can be controlled with drugs, however unwanted side effects usually occur. Drugs are foreign substances to the body and cannot be used as building blocks for more healthy cells.

Cells continually mature and die, only to be replaced by new, young cells. Some cells live days, others live years, but your body is continually regrowing itself. Nutritional therapy does not work so much by healing old diseased cells, as it does by fostering the growth of new healthy cells. After repeated generations of healthy cell replacement, the organ and organism have a greater state of well being. This is the miracle of healing.

Many external factors such as genetics, pollution and adaptation to stress may interfere and delay this process. But, in nearly all known conditions, when there is optimum nutrition, a more rapid and seemingly higher state of health results. Most modern physiology textbooks support this observation. For some reason, this process has been undervalued and overlooked by a large portion of mainstream medicine and their educational institutions.

COMMON AILMENTS

In our clinic, many conditions have been observed to respond favorably, in time, using nutritional supplementation and conservative modalities. In cases of life-threatening conditions, we have acted with the cooperation or supervision of a patient's primary treating physician. The following is a partial outline of those formulations which reliably helped people suffering with known conditions.

Dosages have been omitted due to the variations in individual needs resulting from duration of the condition, age, weight, sex, and severity of the problem. Seek a nutritionally minded physician if you feel uncertain about how much to take. Please keep in mind that everyone is different and that it is increasingly more difficult to find a person having just one abnormality at a time or a flawless health record leading up to their problem. Usually, complicated cases require complete nutritional diagnostic procedures including blood and urine testing, hair trace or toxic mineral analysis, digestive capacity evaluation, assessment of diet habits and of course a health history with a physical exam before recommendations can be custom made. With this understanding in mind, we seek to help you to listen to your body and prove nature as being the real healer.

NOTE - Seek the advice of your nutritionally minded physician (or convert him or her into one) before altering any therapies that your physician has prescribed. If you have been taking prescription drugs, these must usually be discontinued gradually as your body becomes healthy enough to do without the drug. If you quit the drug *cold turkey* without proper planning or guidance this can often provoke a health crisis. Seek the advice of your prescribing physician.

Acne - mild to severe bacterial infection of the skin due to excessive oil production, stress, weakened immune function or hormonal imbalance

> *Multiple vitamin/mineral supplement*
> *Protein powder*
> *Zinc*
> *Herbal laxative formula*
> *Immune support formula*
> *Beta-carotene*
> *Vitamin C*
> *Garlic*

Alcoholism - regular use of alcohol in place of natural methods of stress control

> *Multiple vitamin/mineral supplement*
> *Protein powder*
> *Zinc*
> *Vitamin E with selenium*
> *B-Complex formula*
> *Alfalfa*
> *Vitamin C*
> *Acidophilus or Bifidus*

Allergies - sneezing, itching, congestion, headaches, tiredness, anxiety, rashes

> *Multiple vitamin/mineral supplement*
> *Protein powder*
> *Vitamin C*
> *Calcium*
> *Alfalfa*
> *Immune support formula*
> *Zinc*
> *Garlic*

Anemia - low red blood cell concentration

Multiple vitamin/mineral supplement
Protein powder
Iron
Vitamin C
B-Complex formula
Acidophilus or Bifidus

Angina - chest tightness with pain

Multiple vitamin/mineral supplement
Protein powder
Vitamin E with selenium
Lecithin
Calcium magnesium
EPA or GLA
B-Complex formula
Vitamin C
Garlic

Arteriosclerosis - plugging of the arteries of the heart

Multiple vitamin/mineral supplement
Protein powder
EPA or GLA
Lecithin
Calcium magnesium
Alfalfa
Psyllium fiber
Garlic
Acidophilus or Bifidus

Arthritis - joint pains with or without swelling

Multiple vitamin/mineral supplement
Protein powder
Alfalfa
Calcium magnesium
Herbal laxative formula
Beta-carotene
Lecithin
B-Complex formula
Vitamin C
Zinc
Vitamin E with selenium
Psyllium fiber
Acidophilus or Bifidus

Asthma - bronchial constriction and wheezing due to allergic or stress response

Multiple vitamin/mineral supplement
Protein powder
Vitamin C
Vitamin E with selenium
Zinc
B-Complex formula
Garlic

Broken Bones - fracture, usually caused from an injury

Multiple vitamin/mineral supplement
Protein powder
Alfalfa
Multiple mineral complex
Calcium
Vitamin C
Zinc

Bronchitis - persistent upper chest congestion with painful cough

Multiple vitamin/mineral supplement
Protein powder
Beta-carotene
Immune support formula
Vitamin C
Herbal laxative formula
Garlic

Bursitis - progressive pain in shoulder, elbows, hips, or knees

Multiple vitamin/mineral supplement
Protein powder
Herbal laxative formula
Vitamin E with selenium
Vitamin C
Psyllium fiber
Acidophilus or Bifidus

Cancer Prevention - uncontrolled growth of abnormal cells

Multiple vitamin/mineral supplement
    or
Liquid Vitamin/Mineral Supplement
Protein powder
Herbal laxative formula
Vitamin C
Beta-carotene
Zinc
B-Complex formula
Lecithin
Vitamin E with selenium
Immune support formula
Acidophilus or Bifidus

Candida Yeast - fungal overgrowth of the bowel following antibiotics, stress, improper diet, or prescription drugs

> *Multiple vitamin/mineral supplement*
> *Protein powder*
> *Garlic*
> *Vitamin C*
> *Acidophilus or Bifidus*

Canker Sores - painful blister or lesion on or in mouth

> *Multiple vitamin/mineral supplement*
> *Protein powder*
> *Immune support formula*
> *Vitamin C*
> *B-Complex formula*
> *Beta-carotene*
> *Garlic*
> *L-lysine*

Cataracts - calcium salts clouding lens of eye

> *Multiple vitamin/mineral supplement*
> *Protein powder*
> *Zinc*
> *Vitamin C*
> *Vitamin E with selenium*

Chemical Dependency - habitual use of artificially synthesized drugs

> *Multiple vitamin/mineral supplement*
> *Protein powder*
> *B-Complex formula*
> *Calcium magnesium*
> *Lecithin*
> *Herbal laxative formula*
> *Psyllium fiber*
> *Vitamin C*
> *Acidophilus or Bifidus*

Chronic Fatigue Syndrome - decreased immune function caused by nutrient deficiencies and exposure to viruses and toxins

Multiple vitamin/mineral supplement
Protein powder
Vitamin C
B-Complex formula
Immune support formula
Garlic
EPA or GLA

Colitis - excessive watery bowel movements with or without pain, with or without bleeding

Liquid Vitamin/Mineral Supplement
Protein powder
Alfalfa
Psyllium fiber
Zinc
Acidophilus or Bifidus
Garlic

Common Cold - a viral infection causing chills, fever, sinus congestion, runny nose, fatigue, or sore throat. The common cold normally lasts 7 to 10 days. Early treatment can minimize symptoms and speed your recovery. Drink extra liquids, rest, and minimize food intake with a fever.

Multiple vitamin/mineral supplement
Immune support formula
Protein powder
Vitamin C
Beta-carotene
Zinc
Lecithin
Calcium magnesium
Acidophilus or Bifidus
Garlic

Constipation - reduced frequency of bowel movements (to be healthy, one should have at least two bowel movements daily)

Multiple vitamin/mineral supplement
Protein powder
Herbal laxative formula
Psyllium fiber
Alfalfa
Lecithin
B-Complex formula

Crohn's disease - painful irritable bowel condition involving immune function, circulation, and digestion

Multiple vitamin/mineral supplement
Protein powder
Vitamin E with selenium
Herbal laxative formula
Acidophilus or Bifidus
Zinc
Beta-carotene

Depression - feeling of worthlessness usually accompanied by fatigue, often with loss of appetite

Multiple vitamin/mineral supplement
Protein powder
B-Complex formula
Lecithin

Diabetes - There are two types of diabetes

Adult onset diabetes is the most common type, which is caused by suppression of insulin production due to over-consumption of fats and sugars, stress, or exposure to certain drugs and chemical pollutants.

Juvenile diabetes is caused by a defect in the insulin producing cells of the pancreas. This defect may be genetic, the result of an injury, or a viral infection.

Multiple vitamin/mineral supplement
Protein powder
Alfalfa
Zinc
Lecithin
B-Complex formula
Vitamin E with selenium
Chromium

Eczema - itching or burning lesions of the skin having blisters, scales, crusts or swelling which can be caused by multiple factors

Multiple vitamin/mineral supplement
Protein powder
Herbal laxative formula
Alfalfa
Zinc
Vitamin E with selenium
Immune support formula

Emphysema - hardening of lung membranes caused from pollutants, mainly cigarette smoke, which results in difficulty in emptying the lungs

Multiple vitamin/mineral supplement
Protein powder
Vitamin E with selenium
Vitamin C
Beta-carotene
Alfalfa

Flu - viral infection, often with fever and depression, affecting digestion, muscles, nose, and nervous system

> *Multiple vitamin/mineral supplement*
> *Protein powder*
> *Vitamin C*
> *Vitamin E*
> *Lecithin*
> *Immune support formula*
> *Calcium*
> *Beta-carotene*

Glaucoma - increased pressure in the eye due to increased fluid pressure within the eye. Usually found in the elderly, it may cause blindness if untreated.

> *Multiple vitamin/mineral supplement*
> *Protein powder*
> *Vitamin E with selenium*
> *Beta-carotene*
> *Vitamin C*
> *Zinc*
> *Alfalfa*
> *Herbal laxative formula*

Headaches - a diffuse pain in different portions of the head (there are many types and causes of headaches)

> *Multiple vitamin/mineral supplement*
> *Protein powder*
> *Alfalfa*
> *B-Complex formula*
> *Lecithin*
> *Calcium*

Heart Disease - disorders that develop from malnutrition during development or during times of heavy stress

> *Multiple vitamin/mineral supplement*
> *Protein powder*
> *Psyllium fiber*
> *Vitamin E with selenium*
> *Lecithin*
> *Alfalfa*
> *Vitamin C*
> *Multiple mineral complex*
> *Zinc*
> *B-Complex formula*
> *Acidophilus or Bifidus*
> *Garlic*

Hemorrhoids - swelling, itching or protruding of anal tissue with or without bleeding

> *Multiple vitamin/mineral supplement*
> *Protein powder*
> *Herbal laxative formula*
> *Psyllium fiber*
> *Vitamin E with selenium*
> *Lecithin*
> *B-Complex formula*
> *Vitamin C*
> *EPA*
> *Acidophilus or Bifidus*
> *Garlic*

Hyperactivity - a condition found in children who have reduced attention span and behavioral problems caused by specific vitamin and mineral deficiencies and food or environmental sensitivities

> *Multiple vitamin/mineral supplement*
> *Protein powder*
> *B-Complex formula*
> *Alfalfa*
> *Lecithin*
> *Herbal laxative formula*

Hyperlipidemia - elevated blood cholesterol, LDL or triglycerides

> *Multiple vitamin/mineral supplement*
> *Protein powder*
> *Psyllium fiber*
> *Alfalfa*
> *Lecithin*
> *Acidophilus or Bifidus*
> *Garlic*
> *Herbal laxative formula*

Hypertension - elevated blood pressure measured when at rest

> *Multiple vitamin/mineral supplement*
> *Protein powder*
> *EPA*
> *GLA*
> *Acidophilus or Bifidus*
> *Garlic*
> *Psyllium fiber*
> *Herbal laxative formula*

Hyperthyroidism - excessive release of thyroid hormone, causing weight loss, pounding heart, insomnia, muscle wasting and bulging eyes

> *Multiple vitamin/mineral supplement*
> *Protein powder*
> *Immune support formula*
> *B-Complex formula*
> *Beta-carotene*
> *Garlic*
> *EPA or GLA*

Hypoglycemia - Low blood sugar, a condition made worse by eating too much sugar and refined carbohydrates

> *Multiple vitamin/mineral supplement*
> *Protein powder*
> *Alfalfa*
> *Zinc*
> *Lecithin*
> *B-Complex formula*
> *Vitamin E with selenium*
> *Chromium*

Hypothyroidism - reduced production or inhibition of thyroid hormone, causing fatigue, weight gain, mental confusion, thinning hair and depression

> *Multiple vitamin/mineral supplement*
> *Protein powder*
> *Alfalfa*
> *Calcium magnesium*
> *Vitamin C*
> *Vitamin E with selenium*
> *Zinc*
> *Lecithin*

Insomnia - unable to easily get to sleep, or wake up and can't easily get back to sleep

> *Multiple vitamin/mineral supplement*
> *Protein powder*
> *Lecithin*
> *Calcium*
> *Vitamin C*
> *Acidophilus or Bifidus*

Jaundice - yellow discoloration of skin and whites of the eyes due to faulty liver function

> *Multiple vitamin/mineral supplement*
> *Protein powder*
> *Zinc*
> *Lecithin*
> *Alfalfa*
> *Vitamin E with selenium*
> *Vitamin C*
> *Beta-carotene*
> *Garlic*
> *Acidophilus or Bifidus*

Kidney Stones - salts of calcium, amino acids, uric acid, carbonates or phosphates which are not soluble in urine

> *Multiple vitamin/mineral supplement*
> *Protein powder*
> *Alfalfa*
> *B-Complex formula*
> *Lecithin*
> *Herbal laxative formula*
> *Acidophilus or Bifidus*

Laryngitis - inflammation of the voice box causing hoarseness and raspiness of the voice

> *Multiple vitamin/mineral supplement*
> *Protein powder*
> *Zinc*
> *Vitamin C*
> *Immune support formula*
> *Garlic*

Leg Pains - discomfort in the calves, thighs or top of the feet, especially at night

> *Multiple vitamin/mineral supplement*
> *Protein powder*
> *Alfalfa*
> *Calcium magnesium*
> *Vitamin E with selenium*
> *Acidophilus or Bifidus*

Liver Disorders - metabolic or toxic conditions which reduce normal function of the liver in a number of ways

> *Multiple vitamin/mineral supplement*
> *Protein powder*
> *Herbal laxative formula*
> *Psyllium fiber*
> *Lecithin*
> *Alfalfa*
> *Vitamin E with selenium*
> *Vitamin C*
> *Beta-carotene*
> *Garlic*
> *Acidophilus or Bifidus*

Malabsorption Syndrome - reduced absorption of nutrients due to factors such as stress, hectic lifestyle, allergies, and drug toxicity

> *Multiple vitamin/mineral supplement*
> *Protein powder*
> *Herbal laxative formula*
> *Vitamin C*
> *Lecithin*
> *Alfalfa*
> *Acidophilus or Bifidus*
> *Psyllium fiber*

Menstrual Difficulties - excessive flow, irregular frequency or excessive fatigue

Multiple vitamin/mineral supplement
Protein powder
EPA or GLA
Vitamin E with selenium
B-Complex formula
Alfalfa
Multiple mineral complex

Mental Depression - loss of interest in normally challenging activities with symptoms of lethargy or insomnia

Multiple vitamin/mineral supplement
Protein powder
B-Complex formula
Lecithin
Herbal laxative formula
Acidophilus or Bifidus

Mononucleosis - a delayed immune response in the liver caused by the Epstein-Barr virus (EBV). This condition causes extreme fatigue usually with enlarged lymph nodes. Stress reduction and rest are essential to recovery.

Multiple vitamin/mineral supplement
Protein powder
Vitamin C
Beta-carotene
Garlic
Zinc
Calcium magnesium
Herbal laxative formula
Psyllium fiber

Multiple Sclerosis - failure to remyelinate (insulate) nerves due to past viral infections, genetic weakness and inability to detoxify fat residues in the body. This causes numbness, general muscle weakness, chronic constipation, slurred speech and occasional blindness.

Multiple vitamin/mineral supplement
Protein powder
Lecithin
B-Complex formula
Vitamin E with selenium
Calcium magnesium
Herbal laxative formula
Garlic
Acidophilus or Bifidus
Psyllium fiber

Muscle Pain with Spasm - sudden discomfort and uncontrollable tightening of isolated muscles in the body

Multiple vitamin/mineral supplement
Protein powder
Vitamin E with selenium
B-Complex formula
Calcium magnesium

Nervousness - excitability of the nervous system associated with unrest

Multiple vitamin/mineral supplement
Protein powder
B-Complex formula
Lecithin
Acidophilus or Bifidus

Night Blindness - inability to regain vision in reduced light immediately after leaving a well lighted area

Multiple vitamin/mineral supplement
Protein powder
Beta-carotene

Obesity - weighing more than 20% above ideal weight

> *Multiple vitamin/mineral supplement*
> *Protein powder*
> *Calcium magnesium*
> *Herbal laxative formula*
> *Psyllium fiber*
> *EPA or GLA*
> *Acidophilus or Bifidus*

Osteoporosis - loss of bone density and stature usually in post menopausal women, ultimately resulting in spontaneous fractures

> *Multiple vitamin/mineral supplement*
> *Protein powder*
> *Calcium magnesium*
> *Multiple mineral complex*
> *Alfalfa*
> *Acidophilus or Bifidus*

Pneumonia - bacterial, viral or yeast lung infections which are recurring, or return following antibiotic therapy

> *Multiple vitamin/mineral supplement*
> *Protein powder*
> *Vitamin C*
> *Immune support formula*
> *B-Complex formula*
> *Lecithin*
> *Vitamin E with selenium*
> *Garlic*

Premenstrual Syndrome (PMS) - extreme symptoms of anxiety, irritability, body aches, insomnia and depression

> *Multiple vitamin/mineral supplement*
> *Protein powder*
> *EPA or GLA*
> *Lecithin*
> *Performance*
> *Alfalfa*

Prostatic Enlargement - slow urine flow often with a feeling of urgency commonly occurring in mature men

Multiple vitamin/mineral supplement
Protein powder
Zinc
Vitamin C
Beta-carotene
Alfalfa
Vitamin E with selenium
Lecithin
B-Complex formula
Calcium

Psoriasis - inflamed skin irritation with flaking and reddened patches often associated with arthritic disease

Multiple vitamin/mineral supplement
Protein powder
Alfalfa
Beta-carotene
Herbal laxative formula
Immune support formula
Vitamin C
Vitamin E with selenium
Zinc
B-Complex formula
Protein powder
Calcium magnesium
Acidophilus or Bifidus
Garlic

Sinusitis - inflamed or infected sinuses brought on by allergies or as a residual effect from a virus

Multiple vitamin/mineral supplement
Protein powder
Vitamin C
Immune support formula
Alfalfa
Calcium
Beta-carotene
Garlic

Sore Throat - burning pain of the lining of the throat often with painful coughing

Multiple vitamin/mineral supplement
Protein powder
Beta-carotene
Zinc
Vitamin C
Garlic

Stress - when specialized hormones are released due to threatening situations, survival instincts propel the body toward exhaustion. These nerve hormones cause tense muscles, digestion slows and elimination processes are reduced. Insomnia, body aches & pains, indigestion and fatigue result.

Multiple vitamin/mineral supplement
Protein powder
Vitamin C
Calcium magnesium
B-Complex formula
Lecithin
Alfalfa

Stroke - trauma in the brain caused by a ruptured small artery or a micro blood clot

Multiple vitamin/mineral supplement
Protein powder
Psyllium fiber
Vitamin E with selenium
Lecithin
Herbal laxative formula
Garlic

Tinnitus - a subjective ringing or tinkling sound in the ear

Multiple vitamin/mineral supplement
Protein powder
Zinc
Alfalfa
Beta-carotene
Multiple mineral complex

Tonsillitis - swelling and pain of the tonsils in the back of the throat

Multiple vitamin/mineral supplement
Protein powder
Immune support formula
Vitamin C
Beta-carotene
Zinc
Garlic
Acidophilus or Bifidus

Ulcers of the stomach - stomach pain with bleeding occurring between meals

Multiple vitamin/mineral supplement
Protein powder
Beta-carotene
Zinc
Alfalfa
B-Complex formula
Vitamin E with selenium
Garlic
Acidophilus or Bifidus

Varicose Veins - unsightly swelling with discoloration of the veins on the surface of the legs, ankles and thighs

Multiple vitamin/mineral supplement
Protein powder
Herbal laxative formula
Psyllium fiber
B-Complex formula
Vitamin E with selenium
Garlic

Worms - parasitic infection of the bowel due to the presence of small round worms (pinworms) contracted from pets and causing occasional itching of the anus or grinding of the teeth at night

> *Multiple vitamin/mineral supplement*
> *Protein powder*
> *Herbal laxative formula*
> *Alfalfa*
> *Garlic*
> *Acidophilus or Bifidus*

PERSONAL NOTES

PREVENTIVE NUTRITIONAL SUPPORT

In a more positive light, we should look at the function of supplements (concentrated food) towards healthy conditions.

Pregnancy - This condition is the full blooming of life and not a disease. The metabolism of women increases by approximately 30% during pregnancy and nursing, which increases the need for some essential nutrients well above the normal recommended daily allowances. These are the most important ones we have found.

> *Multiple vitamin/mineral supplement*
> *Protein powder*
> *Alfalfa*
> *B-Complex formula*
> *Vitamin E*
> *Vitamin C*
> *Lecithin*
> *Calcium magnesium*

Early Child Growth - A child's nervous system continues to develop through the first nine months of life. The immune system does not fully mature until puberty. A four year old boy has greater protein needs than his father. Vitamin and mineral catalysts for growth are essential for healthy development and the prevention of chemical imbalances later on in life.

> *Multiple vitamin/mineral supplement*
> *or*
> *Liquid Vitamin/Mineral Supplement*
> *Protein powder*
> *Vitamin C*
> *Calcium magnesium*
> *Multiple mineral complex*
> *Lecithin*
> *Immune support formula*
> *Acidophilus or Bifidus*
> *Garlic*

Athletes - The word *amateur* means *love* of whereas a *professional* does a sport for a livelihood. It has been said that the healthiest people are those that are *amateur* athletes - doing playful and carefree exercise for fun. Rarely do professional athletes stay in top shape after their career. We can all find something we enjoy doing at least 3-5 times a week that raises our heart and respiratory rate. Here is what we need to consider supplementing at all ages to enjoy the sport:

> *Multiple vitamin/mineral supplement*
> *Protein powder*
> *Vitamin C*
> *B-Complex formula*
> *Calcium*

Menopause - The change of life for a woman should be a celebration. The end of the fertility cycle brings new opportunities as well as potential pitfalls. Maintaining activity and productivity requires a woman to be thoroughly aware of her needs after the monthly wave of estrogen is reduced. When hormonal imbalances are present menopause starts as early as the late 30's. Symptoms include dry skin, reduced libido, sagging muscles, headaches, hot flashes. In later stages, stooped shoulders, depression and general fatigue may result. Optimum nutrient balance is essential for this middle age transition.

> *Multiple vitamin/mineral supplement*
> *Protein powder*
> *Beta-carotene*
> *EPA or GLA*
> *Vitamin E with selenium*
> *Vitamin C*
> *Multiple mineral complex*
> *Calcium magnesium*

Old Age - The needs of mature individuals are receiving greater study. If we live as we should when we are young, we won't have to pay the overdue interest on an unhealthy life when we are older. Old age is a misleading statement. We have met people who are in their eighties and getting younger by the year while people in their thirties are aging by the minute. Premature aging is what we would all like to prevent. Maturing is a word I prefer to use more (now that we are grandparents)!

Multiple vitamin/mineral supplement
Protein powder
Vitamin E with selenium
Vitamin C
Psyllium fiber
Calcium magnesium
Multiple mineral complex
B-Complex formula
Lecithin
Garlic
Beta-carotene

PERSONAL NOTES

APPENDIX A

THE ADVERSE EFFECTS OF DRUGS ON NUTRITION

During health crises, some drugs are indeed helpful in giving a person the time needed to implement a healthier nutritional lifestyle. On the other hand, many drugs interfere with the action of nutrients in the body. This outline describes the dangerous effects of taking something to mask symptoms. Almost one half of the patients we see are suffering from drug-induced nutrient deficiencies. We hope this list will be helpful in your support of our motto - *Just Say No to Drugs! Say Yes to Nutrition!*

The following list of commonly prescribed drugs and their effects on vitamin and mineral status is from *Clinical Assessment of Nutritional Status, a Working Manual* by Alan H. Pressman, DC and Alan H. Adams, DC

Drug	Nutritional Interaction	Clinical Significance
Analgesics Non-narcotic salicylates Aspirin	Decreased platelet level of Vitamin C	Can cause hypoprothrom- binemia and lengthen bleeding time
	Iron deficiency	
	Folate deficiency	Increased numbers of deformed babies born to mothers on salicylates
	Malabsorption of glucose	High doses cause GI and xylosedisturbances Can produce GI bleeding, especially with alcohol
Anorexic Agents Amphetamines Benzadrine Dexedrine Desoxyn Dexamil	Decreases appetite Gastric irritant	Suppresses growth in young children
Antacids All antacids	Destruction of thiamin	Occurs mainly with chronic use (i.e., hourly)
	Decrease in absorption of iron	
	Increase in amount of sodium in the body	Can cause fluid retention

Drug	Nutritional Interaction	Clinical Significance
Aluminum Antacids		
Maalox Gelusil Amphojel Mylanta	Decreases absorption of phosphate Decreases the absorption of Vitamin A	May cause hypophosphat-emia, hypercalciuria, hypo-magnesemia, osteomalacia, renal stones
Calcium containing antacids	Decreased absorption of phosphate	May induce constipation Hypophosphatemia
Sodium bicarbonate	Decreased absorption of magnesium Increased sodium in the body Possibly decreased absorption of iron	Can cause steatorrhea or constipation May cause edema Significant only in large doses
Antibiotics		
Amphotericin	Increases the excretion of magnesium, phosphate, potassium	Can cause severe hypo-kalemia, hypomagnesemia, hypophosphatemia
Chloramphenicol	Increases the iron in the serum Decreases folate, Vitamin B12 and hemotopoietic response Decreases absorption of glucose and amino acids	Anemia often seen
Cycloserine	Decreases folate in serum Deficiency of pyridoxine	May see neurological symptoms of pyridoxine deficiency
Ethambutol	Zinc and/or copper metabolism is altered	
Gentamicin Capreomycin Tobramycin Viomycin	Increases the excretion of calcium, magnesium, and possibly phosphate	Severe electrolyte disturbances
Isoniazid	Pyridoxine deficiency	Neuritis which may be incapacitating The malnourished and alcoholics are more susceptible to deficiencies

Drug	Nutritional Interaction	Clinical Significance
Kanamycin Neomycin Paromomycin	Decreases the absorption of Vitamins A, D, K, B12	Can cause significant malabsorption with chronic therapy
	Decreases the absorption of sodium, potassium, iron, calcium	
	Decreases absorption of fat, cholesterol, sugar, protein	
Para-aminosalicylic acid (PAS)	Decreases absorption of B12, folate, cholesterol, xylose	Malabsorption, Megaloblastic anemia
	Decrease in Vitamin K coagulation factors	Only with those patients on anticoagulants
	Increased excretion of potassium	Hypokalemia
	Can cause deficiency of pyridoxine	
Penicillin	Delayed absorption when taken with food	
	May cause malabsorption of Vitamin B12, calcium, magnesium, glucose, carotene and cholesterol	
	May decrease Vitamin K synthesis	
	May decrease folate utilization and inactivates pyridoxine	
Tetracycline	Decreases the absorption of calcium, iron, magnesium, copper, cobalt, manganese, zinc	
	Decreases the Vitamin K dependent coagulation factors	Most common in long-term oral therapy in combination with low dietary intake of Vitamin K. Often seen in patients on anticoagulants.
	Decreases leukocyte ascorbic acid level	
	Can cause deficiency of riboflavin, pyridoxine, Vitamin B12	
	Decreases level of pantothenic acid in serum	
	Can cause weight loss	

Drug	Nutritional Interaction	Clinical Significance
Anticoagulants Sodium Warfarin Coumadin	Decreases Vitamin K dependent factors	The likelihood of a deficiency increases when there is a deficiency of potassium, ascorbic acid and dietary fat
	Prothrombin time decreases if the patient is also taking griseofulvin	
Anticonvulsants Phenobarbital Diphenylhydantoin	Accelerated Vitamin D metabolism	Rickets in children, osteo- malacia in adults
	Decreased calcium absorption	
	Accelerated Vitamin K metabolism	
	Low serum levels of folate, especially after 5 years or more of therapy	Can cause mental distur- bances and neuropathy
	Hypomagnesemia in pileptics who take anticonvulsants	Gastric irritant
	Possible Vitamin B12 deficiency if intake has been low	Effect altered with alcohol
Antidiabetic Agents Insulin		May be teratogenic, no Definite proof if defects are due to nutritional causes
Sulfonylureas Tolbutamide Chlorpropamide Tolazamide Acetohexamide	Malabsorption of xylose, glucose	Gastric irritant Antabuse-like reaction if taken in combination with alcohol
Biguanides Phenformin	Malabsorption of Vitamin B12, calcium, amino acids, glucose, xylose, fat, water electrolytes	Gastric irritant Taste acuity is altered

Drug	Nutritional Interaction	Clinical Significance
Antihyperlipemics		
Colestipol Colestid Cholestyramine Questran	Malabsorption of Vitamins A, D, E, K Decreased absorption of Vitamins A, B12	Constipation can occur
	Decreased absorption of iron, electrolytes, xylose	
	Vitamin K deficiency with prolonged use in high doses	
	Decreases Vitamin K-dependent factors	
Clofibrate Atromid-S	May decrease the absorption of Vitamin B12, iron, carotene, glucose, electrolytes, medium chain trigly- cerides,and xylose	Weight gain Nausea Diarrhea Altered taste senasations
Anti-inflammatory Agents		
Colchicine	Decreases absorption of Vitamins A, D, B12, fat xylose, lactose	
Salicylates	Decreases Vitamin K- dependent coagulation factors	Seen only when used in high doses over a long period of time. Uncommon
Antineoplastics		
Actinomycin D Mithramycin	Decreases absorption of calcium	Hypocalcemia (a desired therapeutic effect of mithramycin)
Cyclophosphamide	Decreases absorption of fat	Can cause severe steatorrhea (although uncommon)
	Decreases absorption of thiamine	
Methotrexate	Causes deficiency of folate	Toxicity is enhanced if there is an existing deficiency of folate and
	Decreased absorption of Vitamin B12, carotene, fat, cholesterol, lactose, xylose	Vitamin B12
Cardiovascular Preparations		
Digitalis Cardiac glycosides Acylanid Digitaline Lanoxin	Increases rate of excretion of calcium, magnesium Decrease in absorption of glucose and xylose	Either hypercalcemia or hypokalemia can induce toxicity
	Magnesium deficiency increases sensitivity to drug	
Nitroglycerin	Hypotension can be induced with consumption of alcohol	

Drug	Nutritional Interaction	Clinical Significance
Corticosteroids Cortisone Prednisone	Increases metabolism of Vitamin D	Can cause accelerated bone loss
	Increased excretion of Vitamin C, zinc, potassium, magnesium	Can cause delayed wound healing (from inadequate zinc) and muscle weakness from inadequate potassium
	Increased need of Vitamin B6	May cause abnormalities of glucose tolerance
Diuretics Chlorothiazide	Increases the excretion of potassium	Can cause muscle weakness
	Increases the excretion of magnesium leading to depletion	Can induce hypoglycemia or aggravate diabetes
	Increased excretion of zinc, iodine	May induce gout
Hypotensives Hydralazine	Can cause Vitamin B6 depletion	Can bring on symptoms of polyneuritis
Laxatives Mineral Oil	Decreases absorption of Vitamins A, D, E, K, and electrolytes	Regular ingestion during pregnancy can cause hypo-thrombinemia
	Decreases absorption of calcium	
Oral Contraceptive Agents	Decreases folate in the serum	Megaloblastic anemia may be seen
	Pyridoxine deficiency	
	Decreased Vitamin B12	Depression, weight gain
	May be increased need for riboflavin	
	Increased plasma Vitamin A, increased serum Vitamin E, increased copper absorption	
	Triglycerides, hemoglobin and hematocrit are increased	

Drug	Nutritional Interaction	Clinical Significance
Parkinsonian Drugs		
Levodopa Dopar	Drug effect reduced by high protein intake	GI disturbances
Larodopa	Pyridoxine interferes with drug action	Possible weight loss and taste changes
	Decreased absorption of glucose, xylose	
Procyclidine Kemadrin		Gastric irritant
Trihexyphenidyl Artane		Gastric irritant Causes dryness in mouth
Sedatives		
Barbiturates Amytal Nembutal Seconal	Increases the requirement for Vitamin C	
	Can cause deficiency of Vitamin D and folate	
	Effect altered with alcohol	

APPENDIX B

HEALTH TALK - Your 24 Hour Telephone
Health and Personal Supplement Advisor

Do you have a question regarding a health problem or nutritional supplement. Check it out! Call Dr. Brouse's 24 hour health advisor with your own touch tone telephone. *HEALTH TALK* is not a cut and dried tape recording. You get individual attention with specific recommendations for your problem. Each profile is unique to your symptom characteristics.

This confidential health service eliminates unnecessary visits to the doctor or hospital emergency room. We encourage people with potentially critical problems to seek help before their condition worsens. Follow these simple steps.

1. Before Calling *HEALTH TALK*, scan the list of 99 topics that are currently available. To reach *HEALTH TALK* call (503) 654-0538.

2. *HEALTH TALK* will ask you to enter the number of the topic you are interested in. *Enter the topic number, pressing one button at a time.*

3. *HEALTH TALK* will name the topic you have called, give a short description of it, and ask if this is the topic you want. If it is, *push the number 1 button on your phone to answer yes.* If it is not the topic you want, *push the number 9 button to answer no,* and *HEALTH TALK* will go back to step 2.

4. Now, just listen to the questions *HEALTH TALK* asks you. *When the answer is yes, press the number 1 button on your phone. When the answer is no, press the number 9 button on your phone.*

Dr. Brouse and Sunnyside Health Center provide HEALTH TALK as a public service and assume no responsibility for the actions or non-actions taken by users of the system. If HEALTH TALK directs you to consult Dr. Brouse regarding your problem call (503) 654-3225 during regular business hours. If you need to order an educational video tape, call our toll-free 24 hour order line (800) 845-2025.

> You must use a touch-tone phone to call *HEALTH TALK*.
> If you don't have one, use a friend's or a public phone.

GENERAL

1. Generally Not Feeling Well
2. Loss of Weight
3. Overweight
4. Difficulty in Sleeping
5. Fever
6. Excessive Sweating
7. Feeling Faint and Fainting
8. Dizziness
9. Headache
10. Cramp
11. Numbness and Tingling
12. Twitching and Trembling
13. Difficulty in Speaking
14. Pain in the Face
15. Hair Loss

SKIN

16. General Skin Problems
17. Facial Skin Problems
18. Swellings Under the Skin
19. Itching Without a Rash
20. Itchy Spots and Rashes
21. Rash with Fever
22. Raised Spots and Lumps

EYES, EARS, NOSE

23. Painful Eye
24. Disturbed or Impaired Vision
25. Earache
26. Noises in the Ear
27. Hearing Loss
28. Runny Nose

MOUTH AND THROAT

29. Sore Mouth or Tongue
30. Toothache
31. Bad Breath
32. Difficulty in Swallowing
33. Sore Throat
34. Hoarseness or Loss of Voice
35. Coughing
36. Coughing Up Blood
37. Wheezing
38. Difficulty in Breathing

STOMACH AND BOWEL

39. Vomiting
40. Frequent Vomiting
41. Abdominal Pain
42. Frequent Abdominal Pain
43. Swollen Abdomen
44. Gas and Belching
45. Diarrhea
46. Constipation
47. Abnormal-looking Bowel Movements

CHEST

48. Palpitations

49. Chest Pains

URINE

50. Abnormally Frequent Urination
51. Abnormal-looking Urine

52. Painful Urination
53. Lack of Bladder Control

NECK, BACK AND ARMS

54. Painful or Stiff Neck
55. Backache

56. Painful Arm or Hand
57. Painful Shoulder

LEGS AND FEET

58. Painful Leg
59. Painful Knee
60. Painful Ankles

61. Swollen Ankles
62. Foot Problems

MIND AND EMOTIONS

63. Confusion
64. Impaired Memory
65. Disturbing Thoughts & Feelings
66. Depression

67. Anxiety
68. Hallucinations
69. Nightmares
70. Strange Behavior

MEN

71. Painful or Enlarged Testicles

72. Painful Intercourse

WOMEN

73. Pain or Lumps in the Breast
74. Breast Problems in New Mothers
75. Absent Periods
76. Heavy Periods Women
77. Painful Periods
78. Lower Abdominal Pain in Women

79. Irregular Vaginal Bleeding
80. Abnormal Vaginal Discharge
81. Vaginal Irritation
82. Abnormal Hairiness in

83. Painful Intercourse

70

COUPLES

84. Failure to Conceive

CHILDREN

85. Crying in Infants
86. Vomiting in Infants
87. Diarrhea in Infants
88. Skin Problems in Infants
89. Fever in Infants
90. Waking at Night
91. Slow Weight Gain

92. Swellings in Children
93. Fever in Children
94. Abdominal Pain in Children
95. Itching in Children
96. Coughing in Children
97. Limping in Children

SENIORS

98. Incontinence in the Elderly

99. Confusion in the Elderly

GET YOUR OWN PERSONALIZED
NUTRITIONAL REPORT

♦ Would you like to know which nutritional supplements and how much are right for you?

♦ Are you taking too much of one supplement and not enough of another?

♦ Would you like an *objective* analysis of your health status using standard blood and urine tests?

♦ Would you like a written explanation *in English* of the meaning of the high or low values in your lab tests?

♦ Would you like to maximize your nutritional well being?

For many people, taking nutritional supplements is a matter of guess work. They may have heard (or even read in this booklet) that a particular supplement helps a certain health condition. Usually the advice proves correct, and the health condition does improve. However, often the results are less than complete. This is because, the individual has never had a *comprehensive* evaluation.

Sunnyside Health Center offers such a comprehensive evaluation. We take the lab test values from standard blood and urine testing that can be performed by your doctor. You send us a copy of the lab report along with your answers to a lifestyle and symptom questionnaire. We take this information and use a sophisticated computer program to analyze your nutritional status and deficiencies. You receive a 20 page report that explains what your lab test results mean and makes recommendations about which nutritional supplements you need, as well as any lifestyle changes that will help you achieve optimum health. Our purpose is to give you a specific nutritional program to follow while teaching you more about yourself.

As an individual reading this booklet, you will find that this personalized nutritional report will help you with your own health. Call or write Sunnyside Health Center today at (503) 654-3225, for a *Build a Better You* packet which contains the questionnaire and laboratory request forms needed to have an evaluation performed, or to schedule a Seminar date.

TELEPHONE CONSULTATION WITH DR. BROUSE

If you have any personal health questions or questions regarding any of the information in this booklet or the use of nutritional supplements, Dr. Brouse is available for telephone consultations.

To schedule a time for your telephone consultation, call Sunnyside Health Center at (503) 654-3225.

DR. BROUSE'S VIDEO TAPES:

Produced before live audiences, each presentation is unique in the most current information and practical advice for making health decisions. No where is there this much knowledge available on video tape that is directed to the preventive-minded person interested in using nutritional supplementation. Taking charge of your own health means having the understanding and wisdom to be your best doctor. Knowing your options will set you free to choose your health future instead of taking the chance of developing disease. Share with a friend and enlighten their thinking.

For a free catalog of the titles and program synopsis call (503) 654-3225. A few of the titles available are:

Acne	Hyperactivity
Alcoholism	Hypertension
Allergies	Hypoglycemia
Anemia	Immune system
Arthritis	Kidneys
Back pain	Liver and gall bladder
Cancer	Malabsorption
Candida yeast	Menopause
Circulation	Metabolic exhaustion
Colitis	Multiple sclerosis
Colon health	Osteoporosis
Crohn's disease	Potassium and health
Depression	Premenstrual syndrome
Detoxification	Prostate
Diabetes	Relaxation
Digestion	Skin care
Fatigue	Stress
Glaucoma	Tension control
Headaches	Viral infections
Healthy hearts	Vitamin C
Hemorrhoids	Women's health

These quality video tapes are in the VHS format only.